NURSING THE
MIND MATTERS II
AUTHOR/JUSTIN
JOHNSON
We have authored
Criminal Minds
Matter, and the Mind
Matters, all available
on amazon and
Barnes & noble.

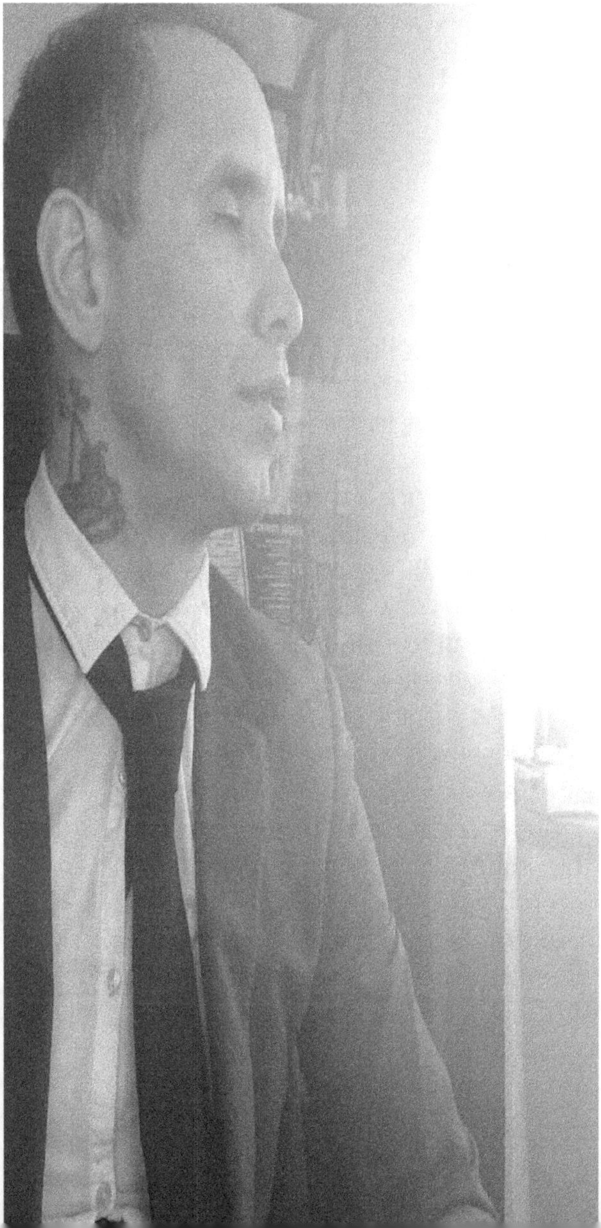

1

Justin D Johnson

Understanding Mental Health First Aid & Mental Health advocacy in the workplace.

Exploring mental health

.

After discovering The Mind Matters first edition, I had decided to look deeper into Mental Health to help support those suffering.

I begun studying with Bath College, as previously suggested I have suffered through Secondary Reynard's Disease Phenomenon and a head injury both illnesses together which gave me anxiety and depression, the depression mainly come's seasonally through the cold weather and lack of sleep. With the first part of this book, I shall produce what I have learnt through my studies of Mental Health and Mental Ill Health, unfortunately many sufferings may not acknowledge their deterioration of their Mental Health or Mental Ill Health which time they receive support or help, it may take more time and forbearance for them to become well again. In some cases, the damage can be forever lasting. You shall learn the different terms of Mental Ill Health & Mental Health and I shall be explaining the definitions of each example. I would like to include that I am also an alienated father and currently in a legal process of divorcing my ex-wife, being away from my children has been a huge impact to my welfare and current state of affairs, but to optimise my full potential I have discovered reading, writing and Art work to become very therapeutic which engages with various varieties of different audiences, even such as athleticism enthusiasts, working class, inequalities the different diverse and ability's hoping to engage with them and also source referencing in such of a way which they may like to engage with everyday activities.

We will be looking at different ways to help prevent Mental Health & Mental Ill Health, such as vitality, health & nutrition, varies of exercises we can do to keep our mind & body's motivated both with examples and guidelines. I will be basing the audience to beginners, for home exercise simple steps that can define your body and mind as an athlete, everything we do, eat, sleep, drink water and exercise, we need to do repetitive and methodical each day. Basic Mental Health steps to prevent us from deteriorating is learning to live with ourselves, sometimes by ourselves. Living independently, we learn to live with what works best, you learn to cook for yourself when your hungry, you learn to drink water when you are thirsty, so you generally get up and do it. Now take this perspective in a civil relationship when one becomes reluctant to wait on their partner to cook or make them a cuppa tea when their thirsty. Everything then seems too mundane it's like they become reliant on their partner to support them. In long marriages let's describe this as our

The Mind Matters ii:

grandparents, nan & grandad. You shall notice one supports the other the most, cooking, cleaning, fetching the cuppa teas, drinks etc. When one of them separate through death of old age or terminally ill health the other usually follows not far behind, weather that be broken hearted or times of lonesome becomes a terrible hardship. Possibly when they start to deteriorate from looking after their own health & hygiene. The morality of bearing a relationship or family weather that be father or mother, boyfriend, or girlfriend, we tend to forget ourselves, our Mental Health, Mental ill Health our wants and needs. Is it a case of noting down to daily remind ourselves that we are important just as they are? Ideally in a civil relationship we shouldn't have to keep reminding ourselves, the ideology relationship should relate right? It should be no other than amicable and reciprocated. Love and marriage is a hard thing to live with, as through thick and thin your supposed to support one another through the good times and the hard times.

It's not just about acknowledging our own mental health, Safeguarding and understanding everyone around us weather that be at work, in a community gathering, art gallery, cinema, church place, being understanding, mindful and being a empath. I mean sometimes if you're with your family, wife, kids or elderly parents we sometimes have to do what's necessarily to protect our loved ones, but always best to be mindful. As attacking someone with mental health weather that be through drunkenness or narcotic abuse can antagonize the mental ill

The Mind Matters ii:

health individual more, which then will leave you into a victim of crime. Many people turn to alcohol weather that be through bereavement, homelessness or break of a marriage etc. Us as humanitarian are the worst culprits to become judges within society. Call safeguarding or local police to advise them they need to make yours and other individuals safety paramount within the area of the mental ill health person or persons. Being mindful and obedient of someone's Mental health or Mental ill health and to acknowledge and support will always improve that person suffering from felling of self-destruct or self-isolated, being arrogant and disobedient of one's Mental health or Mental ill health will be the cause of a series of other implications to ones deterioration of Mental health, such as depression, anxiety then form them to fall into self-destruction, lack of self-care, the lack of feeling loved, loss of sleep, lack of hygiene.

Acknowledging Mental Health & Mental Ill health, Action Plan, Providing Individuals with a support network, So they do not feel isolated or to become a victim of bullying. As you will gather through reading the course of the book, we will see how many within society will polarize against those suffering from Mental Health rather then try to support them, the victim will become then alienated and a victim of being bullied. Each and everyone of us throughout life will face some form of Mental Health deterioration weather that be from bereavement, stress at work, relationship, or debt worries. What we can do is, helpfully advise to vitalize our wellbeing with a good nutrition idea, exercise plan, or just even offer your friend a brisk walk down the beach. Having plenty of rest, sleep and help improve Mental Health struggles. One thing we cannot do is try to understand or mitigate what your friend with Mental Health is going through, because we are all individuals and suffer different circumstances and struggles differently. 'For instance I may not be traumatised from a break up marriage more or less then someone else who is going through the same thing' so let's not patronize others in the frame.

Now we shall begin to define to what is meant by mental health and mental ill health? And we how can we acknowledge, observe those of whom are struggling?

6

PROGSART

Paintings

Mental health:

A person mental and emotional health. It can be positively or emotionally affected and lead to mental disorders A person who has a positive sense who they are and can cope with the normal stresses of life and able to make sense of life and the World around you, think clearly, solve problems, and make sound decisions. Work productively and fruitfully and able to contribute to the community. (Mental Health) The ability to function and deal with everyday life. (Mental Health) A state of well-being in which the individual releases their own abilities, experiencing, understanding and express emotions

The Mind Matters ii:

and feelings. Able to make relationships participate in society!

Some formalised evidence based around the inequalities around us within society, people who suffer, food shortages, excessive bills struggle and worry, the rise of energy cost, fuel prices. These are all added stress to individuals and those who are in relationships or marriages which can tend to lead to break downs and separations. Even those who are in work in a full time but basic paye, working 40+ hours a week, seem to find they're just about covering their bills, rent, water rates, energy supplies, council tax, travel expenses to work, monthly, weekly shopping with very little to have a life outside of work. Those people can work all their lively hood without having a life outside of work or nice fancy cars or holiday trips abroad. Leaving these polarised celebrities on tv or in magazines make our own life's feel estranged and not so important, with their flash cars, big houses, nice clothes, hair, makeup, beautiful excursions, or holidays destinations. When we are lucky to get a free holiday from the Sun newspaper.

(The absence of some or all of these positive factors on an ongoing basis is Mental Ill Health)

The Mind Matters ii:

8

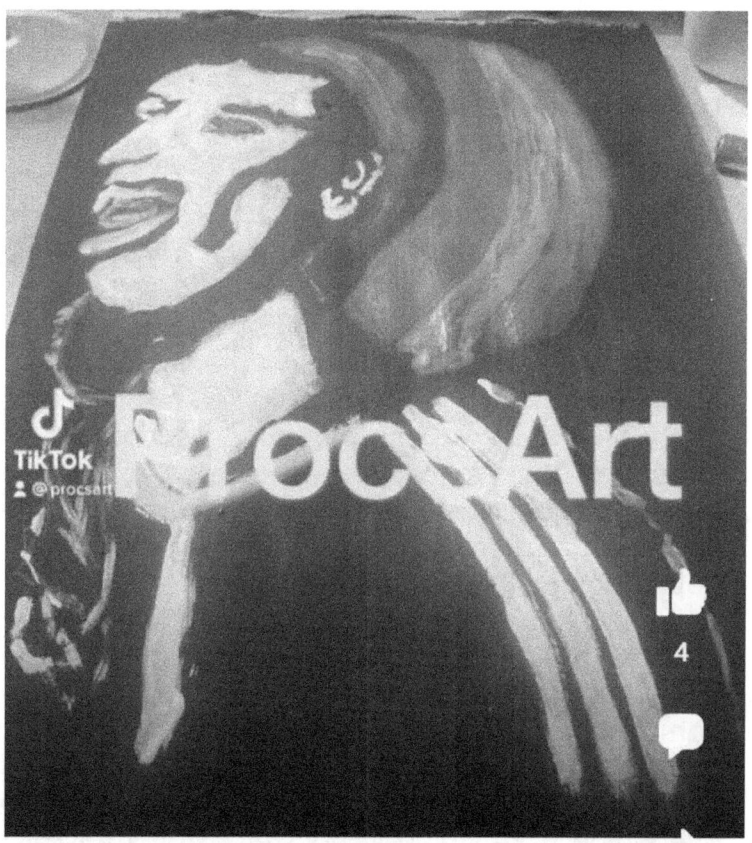

(Bob Marely Impressionist art work)

Mental ill health:

A term that describes both mental illness and mental health problems, affecting those who suffer from both. Mental ILL Health conditions affect, an individual's mood, thinking and behaviour, schizophrenia, and addictive behaviour. (Mental ill Health) anxiety disorder, any condition that disrupts any individual's everyday life, depression.

A massive contribution to Mental ill Health, can be from neglection, a break up from family's, parents or close family your wife or husband, a big factor also is alcoholism and narcotics, a chemical imbalance can trigger many mental ill health disorders, anxiety, schizophrenia, also any trauma many have suffered and can suffer, such as rape, abuse, violence, ex-military, ex athletes, ex fireman, ex doctor, ex police force, nurse surgeons, bus driver, etc.. more than likely anything serving the public domain. I should imagine seeing children being abused, men and women also, it all must have an after effect on one's health both mentally and physically. As we are all empaths and show compassion otherwise, we wouldn't be doing our job specifications. With safeguarding now in every workplace or community halls or gatherings everything or anything is possible. Anyone is also subject to being bullied as we have witnessed in various of newspapers, using safeguarding for their own benefit rather then its actual formal course, a lady just previously calling Essex police of 10 false rape allegation claims against two men, but luckily, they later found evidence she was lying and sentenced to imprisonment. Imagine being one of those innocent men facing these charges at first knowing your innocence? I can guarantee their

The Mind Matters ii:

Mental health or Mental ill health would've deteriorated. Both men had been taken into custody and had their property seized and searched.

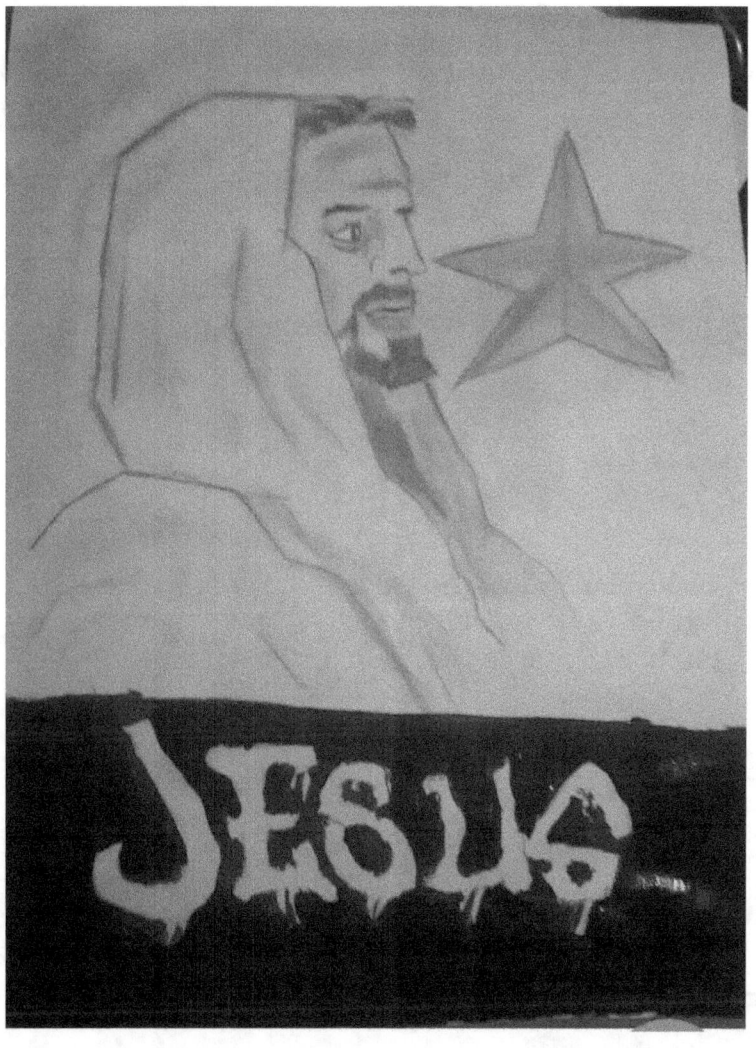

The Mind Matters ii:

what is meant by the mental health continuum.

Let's look at other define factors of the Mental Health continuum, which is the area of mental health & mental illness are at the extremes, depending on a person's inner our outer capabilities. They can change position at any point in the continuum at any time as the situation improves or worsens. Mental health can be thought of a scale that moves from healthy to ill. Everyone's mental health is somewhere along the scale of continuum.

Let's focus from a social scientist perspective through many different factors that may increase the risk of mental ill health in individuals; and, Factors from inside the learning or work environment:

Certain environmental factors have been linked to mental illness. For example, studies show that exposure to certain toxic metals has been linked to various mental disorders. With other factors including fetal development, certain infections, poor nutrition toxins. and other biological environmental factors can lead to mental illness as well.

Inside factors Health & Safety policies are missing or inadequate.

*Poor communication-in work or learning environment which makes individuals not feeling supported.

*Inflexible working/studying hours. They do not support individuals in managing work/life balance

*Unclear tasks.

*Giving individuals tasks which are unsuitable-which may lead to non-achievement of objectives

*High or unrelating workloads or study requirements which mean individuals do not have time to complete tasks

You may also find some individuals have found with trauma they've faced throughout their life; some best find working away from others in their own environment. At their own accord working with a guidance booklet or module books rather than being told, a subject to being vulnerable through a tragic, bullied, brutal attack, beaten, victim of knife crime or

The Mind Matters ii:

rape. Will impact each individual different and not feel safe around others.

Factors from outside the learning or work environment: weather the cause outside of work is sickness, divorce or bereavement or some other trauma the first place is to make sure the workplace is not a stress to the trauma maybe causing anxiety or depression. Could be your wife or husband isn't feeling great at home for example, had an operation causing you a distress whilst at work.

Let's clarify an examples how physical health can affect mental health. We could consider the following factors.

Physical activity and being outdoors:

The body's physical health & Mental health is interconnected, and one cannot be separated from the other, as one affects the other.
A performance of mentally fatigued to a difficult exercise test caused participations to reach exhaustion more quickly when they did the same exercise when mentally rested. Let's base the example's on a physical week at work, gardening for this instance, re-turfing the grass surface, lots of grass shovelling, and top soil, pushing wheel barrow, lot's of cardio, a 9-5 weekly job, building a cardio exercised sweat, throughout the week

The Mind Matters ii:

14

you've built up strength and cardio which your body goes into a cardio pilot mode, following week you don't have a physical job from your 9-5 which is' let's say driving machinery for this instance, a (360 Excavator taking up a driveway) for a patio to be re-laid, you have now found that doing less cardio, but by the time you get home you've found yourself restless and not being able to rest or sleep. It's important to define the difference between the two to, understand how our bodies regulate.

So, it's important to rest up' with peace and mindfulness before a big physical day. is more likely to help you through the day, Sleep, rest, keeping our bodies fuelled such as hydrated, the right nutrition based around the exercise taken place, such as a cardio based, running, cycling, carbohydrates will be more beneficial as slow burning energy is needed. Such as a sprint, or weight lifting explosive exercise protein based diet is more essential, obviously we need to mimic our diet and have a variety of ingredients, carbs, proteins, fats, etc.. But one more then the other depending on exercise we are carrying out.

*Individuals vulnerability- such as low self-esteem and insecurity or inadequate coping mechanisms.

*Lifestyle choices, alcohol or drug use which can put individuals at risk of developing mental health problems

The Mind Matters ii:

*Family history or mental ill health, which may be hereditary

*Problems at home such as domestic violence, neglect, divorce, or family breakdown.

*Feeling cut off- from family and friends or from local community which can lead to feeling of isolation or rejection.

*Negative or traumatic life experiences-such as employment, homelessness, bereavement, sudden illness or being assaulted or abused.

*Big life changes- even where these are positive such as getting married, having children, or moving home which can be stressful for individuals.

*Financial worries-arising unemployment, redundancy business failure, mounting debt or worries about the rising cost of living.

16

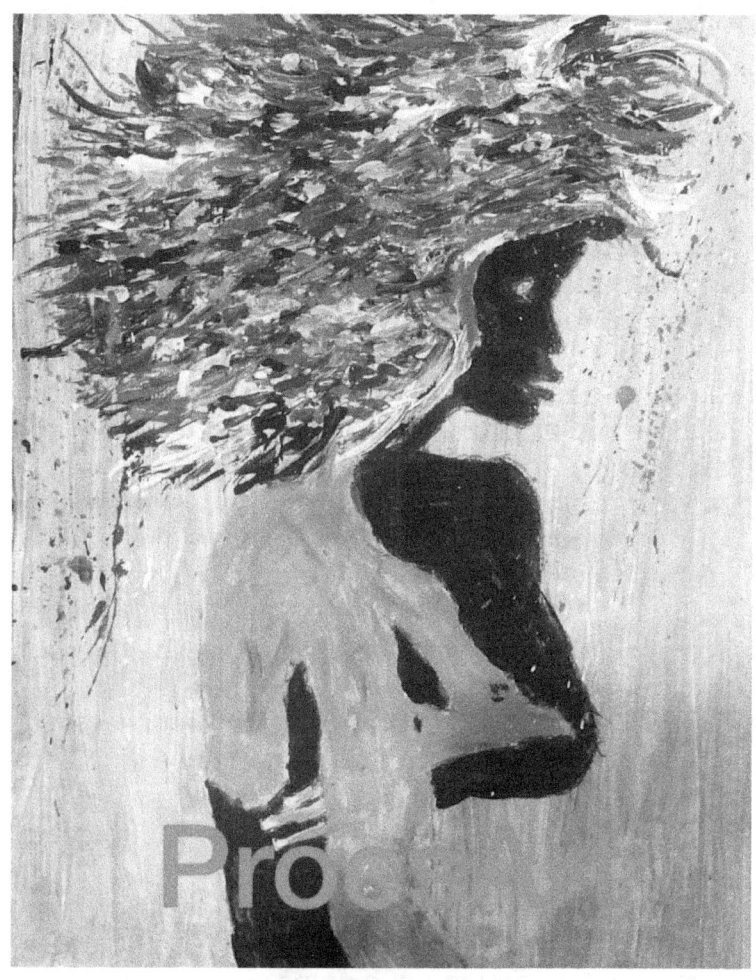

Afrikaans Inequalities impressionist artwork

Nutrition:

The Mind Matters ii:

(Our nutrition benefits) our Vitality is important to us. What we eat is so very important, more important than you think as we tend to eat literally anything when we become starving, such as chocolate, takeaway, crisps etc, these foods I class as rich foods, non-essential food supplies are full of exaggerated fats, sugars and salts, too many carbohydrates also can leave us feeling bloated. Understanding the importance of diet and general nutrition helps us to understand how our mood can vary from a simple diet plan, which can help us feel more energetic, were as a bad diet can make us feel lethargic/sluggish. Our output and altitude on our very own reflection on ourselves is best defined in how we nourish ourselves.

Nutrition affects Mental health and wellbeing, as it promotes and maintains healthy brain development in children and young people. Mental health and nutrition are linked, healthy eating helps young people & children cope more effectively with stress, to better manage their emotions and get a good night's sleep.
Sleep is very efficient for not being fatigued physically and both mentally. The intake of food has an affect on the development of our day-to-day maintenance of our bodies. A balanced diet will help us keep our body healthy which provides the proteins, vitamins, minerals, and other elements our body requires to maintain and repair itself. It's known some deficiencies (of some

The Mind Matters ii:

certain vitamins) can affect our mood and poor diet can leave people feeling tired and lethargic. This will lead is feeling low within our mind set and mood.

As bad nutrition & lack of sleep shows that it can fatigue our moods, generate distress cause anger, how we act and speak to other individuals.

Healthy lifestyle:

Living purely of the ascetics of life will play a massive partial part in our Mental Health and Wellbeing, a better more focused ideology and easier for us to adapt change in how we want to act and what we want to achieve. Intoxication shall add pressure and deteriorate our mental health & wellbeing, also becoming more fatigued and unhealthier. Our lifestyle can depend on our hobbies and interests, and our social circle who we like to participate with.
Such as going to the movies, theatre, Church, attending art galleries, going for walks with family and friends, reading, writing, artwork, playing an instrument.
More society who suffer from worst Mental health or Mental ill health haven't yet sacrificed the worst habits, such as going to a bar, a club, ordering takeaways, salty saturated fats, such as Kentucky, burger king, mac Donald's, kebab shops etc, these are some of the highest forms of intoxication to our body's, It's important we

**notify key elements which need to change to be
sacrificed to better our Mental Health, to our
wellbeing and mental stability, how can we
improve,
Is it our lifestyle, do we need to sacrifice our
friends, is it helping what we eat? Ask
yourselves do I or we need to change?**
Lifestyle, eating healthy, exercising regularly.
getting enough sleep and avoiding harmful levels of
alcohol and drugs can help you keep your mental
health on track. Also manage symptoms of
depression and anxiety and improve your overall
wellbeing. Narcotics and Alcohol and smoking, has
an impact on our mood and Mental Well-being.
Although they will make you happier for a short
while, which will make you feel very low when the
effects wear off and long-term excessive use of
narcotics and alcohol can lead to Mental Health
issues.

Nicotine which is in cigarettes has been shown to
interfere with levels of Dopamine in the brain which
can switch of the brans mechanism for making
Dopamine. Dopamine is a chemical which supports
positive feeling's so lack of it may cause
depression.

**We all need to focus on those around us who
are in our circle, are they our friends? Are these
people a good benefit factor to our Mental
health & well-being? Do they smoke? Do they
drink alcohol take narcotics? Do they have**

The Mind Matters ii:

aggressive mannerism? All these can have a detrimental effect on our mentality on how we end up proposing our aura. Work with what benefit us, what inspires us, what encourages us and who brings out the best in us, (anyone & everyone can change) but we must acknowledge our wrong doings that stop our functioning of human development. We need to make sacrifices from those people who do not benefit from us from bettering our mental health & vitality, from those so-called friends that recognise our mental health problems and ask us to participate within their antics of alcoholism or narcotics anything that can justify a chemical imbalance isn't looking after our vitality. This will have a common defect within bettering our health. You need to plan, visualise what will work best for you to build your prosperous future existence.

Rest/sleep:

how does rest/sleep help improve your mental wellbeing? Rest/sleep helps improves our vision, our focus it also changes our outlook and how we act throughout society. Improves your memory, sharpens your attention. You've probably noticed the more tired you are, the more difficult it is for you to concentrate on anything.

The Mind Matters ii:

Lack of sleep and rest will give us a negative outlook and impact how we look at society, with a less focus and cause complications in how we act in society. So much lack of sleep can cause hallucinations, this could deter in becoming forgetful or even possibly think people in society are starring at you or even laughing which may then cause a sudden distress of a anxiety attack, a common cause of feeling angered, then may lead to start shouting at one another.

Lowers your stress levels, have you ever noticed how the smallest of things bother you if you haven't slept for long enough the night before? Our body needs to repair itself, lack of sleep causes memory issues, puts pressure on the body and can also make people unwell. It's possible to lead to issues with memory and thinking processes, it can cause people to become irritable and behave in such ways of out of character, and trigger anxiety and depression. We also must be ultra-careful when we come to think of operating a vehicle under the influence of sleep deprivation, or operating machinery at work, can be the common cause of a fatal accident waiting to happen

Have you now noticed sleep is highly important in how we reflect on ourselves, of which is determined in our sleep or lack of sleep.

Long-term health conditions:

The Mind Matters ii:

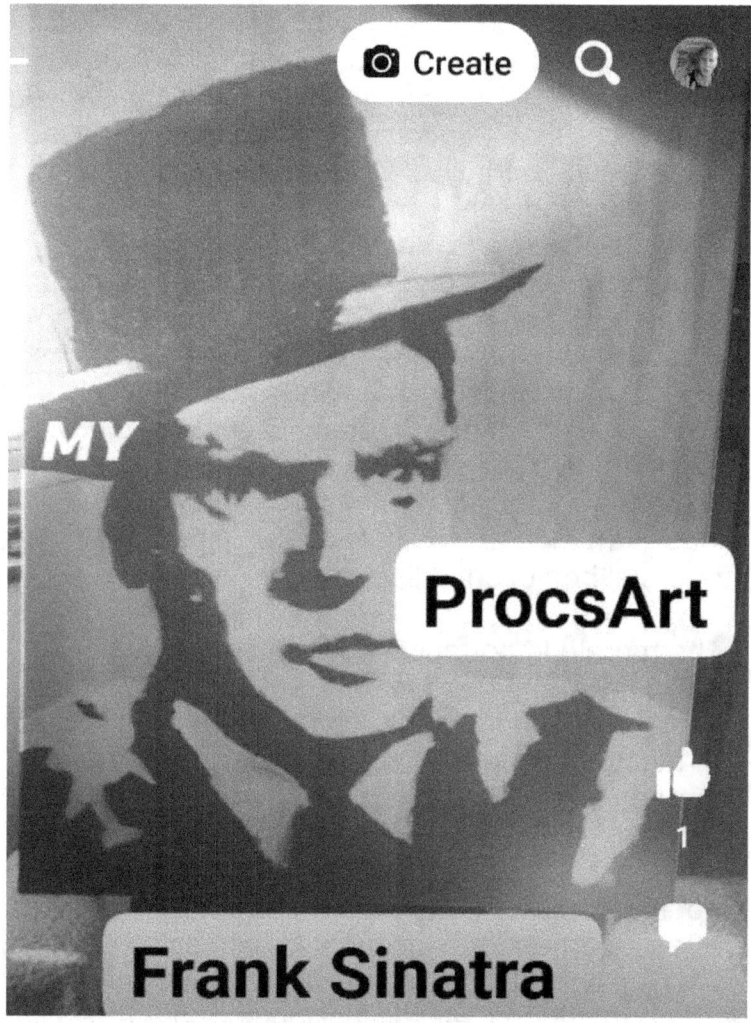

<u>Long Term Health Conditions!</u>

The Mind Matters ii:

Examples of long-term health conditions include diabetes, high blood pressure, arthritis, epilepsy, asthma, and some mental health conditions, if you have more than one long term health conditions this is 'multi-morbity'. These long-term conditions can affect your job. Family and Finances.
However, there are many sources of support.
Long-term health conditions, even where there are not life threatening or life shortening, can lead to Mental Health problems, such as skin conditions like psoriasis which can cause embarrassment, distress, and anxiety. In many cases, people with these types of conditions will not see a Counsellor as part of their treatment plans but may develop long-term Mental-Health issues alongside a physical health condition.

The morale importance of having empathy towards a society that suffer Mental Health and Mental ill health as each individual can suffer from different forms of struggles, weather that be concluded through alcoholism, narcotics, domestic violence, domestic abuse, breakdown of family, friendships, relationships, money management, poor upbringing, the struggle through society with lack of engagement of education, low on opportunities, with different classes of society can proact less unfortunate inequalities, lacking support, now throughout many parts of the UK offer Governmental formed organisations such as alcoholics anonymous, drug addiction help, Peabody money management, debt relief. But first

The Mind Matters ii:

and foremost, identifying what significant steps can you alter first to better your wellbeing and vitality, taking each step carefully to give you a better chance to make adaptations to your health. Like we suggested before this may not be the case for all individuals with Mental health & Mental ill health patients as many suffers can be caused by specific trauma, such as domestic violence or domestic abuse, rape victim, knife victim or even a victim of a highspeed car crash for instance. Any serious cases can lead to frightening through lack of sleep, delusions, hallucinations, disorganised thoughts, slurred speech, and strange behaviour

Our evidence which describes the different types of mental ill health along the continuum. Within our description, it will show you **FIVE** different examples of mental ill health:

1)Schizophrenia, a mental order characterized by delusions, hallucinations, disorganised thoughts, speech, and behaviour.
2) Major depressive disorder, Mental health disorder having episodes of psychological depression
3) bipolar disorder. a serious mental illness characterized by extreme mood swings, they conclude extreme excitement episodes or extreme depressive feelings.

The Mind Matters ii:

4) Post traumatic stress disorder, a mental health condition that develops followed by a traumatic event characterized by the intrusive thoughts about the incident, recurrent distress/anxiety.
5)Autism spectrum disorder, A neurodevelopment disorder that causes a wide range of impairments in social communication and restricted and repetitive behaviours.

Physical health	phycological	behavioural
Changes in appetite.	Mood changes.	Being irritable, angry or aggressive.
Complaining of joint or back pain.	Indecision	Over-reacting to situations
	Appearing sad or low	withdrawal.
Headaches.		
Weight loss or gain	Appearing anxious or distressed	Over excitement
		Increased or excess smoking and drinking.
Indigestion or other stomach complaints	Irrational or illogical thought processes	
Unexplained tiredness.		A resigned attitude
Complaining of not being able to sleep.		Drug taking.
		Repetitive speech or activity

Steps to support individual facing a mental health crisis	What to do is someone is sui
Asking what would help them and being reassuring	Reassure them they are love Call 999 or 101 for emergenc professional help if need be.

The Mind Matters ii:

Listening to them without making any judgements Signposting them to practical information where appropriate, Concentrating on their immediate needs such a dealing with any wounds they might have. Avoiding confrontation. Ask if you can contact someone for them. Encouraging them to seek for help from a crisis team, their GP or other appropriate Professional If they are seeing or hearing things reminding them that you are there and not dismissing their experiences or reinforcing them	

The Mind Matters ii:

Researching the importance of positive relationships and effective communication when supporting individuals with mental ill health;

The importance of positive relationships:

Let's start by explaining a relationship with workers at work how communication support mental health outcome or depleting it, the psychosocial hazards related to culture within an organization, such as poor interpersonal relations lack of practices related to respect for workers are a significant contributor to workplace   stress.

Whilst prolonged exposure to these psychosocial hazards is related to increased psychiatric and psychological health problems, positive social relationships among employees is how work gets done. The importance is composure how employees correspond to their workers, this instance being a nice calm, but persuasive employee will get a lot more from his workforce, to whereas a tired, fatigued miserable employee shall get less work done from his employee as his approach doesn't show any kind of enthusiasm towards his workforce. The destructive annoyance for work colleagues as an employer brings his home life problems, weather that be relationship or money management into their workplace environment can a negative implication in how they manager

The Mind Matters ii:

becomes less self-aware of how he acts irrational towards his working colleagues

The importance of communication:

If you don't ask, you don't speak then the answer will always be a no. The importance of communication at work is very important as one may need a hand to hold something whilst the over operates their task using machinery or a basic hand drill.

Understanding, to make sure you clearly express your wants, your intentions and needs which you can benefit great from within life,

Strengthening relationships, speaking aloud and confident in life are usually the ones that make it the furthest throughout life.
relieving stress
increasing confidence & happiness

The Mind Matters ii:

Understand how to support individuals with mental ill health

The Understanding from the characteristics of a positive relationships.

Throughout a Positive relationship it is important in preventing and supporting Mental Ill Health within all aspects of life, including the workplace, Many full-time workers do spend more time and work within the week rather than with their family & friends.
Being in a negative environment for this large amount of time could cause stress and make individuals feel isolated, which shall reduce motivation and lead to low morale.

It also does have a negative effect on Mental Health an also on productivity at work,

To utilise a better formal stability of Mental Health for a better relationship in a workplace, or even partner it's important to take rest breaks, having a break away from either can make the heart grow fonder, repair as we can become depleted from putting all our motivation into either source, 'work or relationship,' with sometimes not appreciating all the benefits that come from either.

Positive relationships key concepts: 1)Trust 2) Empathy 3) Respect 4) Flexibility 5) Appreciation 6)Reciprocation

The Mind Matters ii:

A positive relationship in a workplace or relationship can best be understood that you are a sufferer of Mental Health or Mental ill Health and to become accepted, which you then can build an understanding of trust and respect, having flexibility to take time out, showing them reciprocation to put the work in on return, this will provide appreciation from either participant.

Our outlook at ways to support an individual with mental ill health for each of the areas identified;

Early intervention:

Tutor, Colleagues, Managers within the workplace or learning environment can play an important part in early intervention to prevent Mental Health decline. They should be able to identify early signs with individuals who are stressed, or their Mental Health is declining. Individuals should be encouraged to talk about their problems that they have at work, from learning or other aspects of the environment.

How can a tutor, Colleague or Manager acknowledge someone's Mental Health decline? As getting to know the person's usual aura and characteristics you will have a general idea on how their mood digests, the more you get to know that person the more you shall grasp an idea to what

The Mind Matters ii:

antagonizes their Mental Health in the workplace, then to offer them support, a break or even time off if   necessary.

With identifying potential problems early, encouraging individuals to talk and understand what support is available, Colleagues, tutors or Managers may be able to help prevent Mental Health decline.

Short-term support:

In short term, talking to individuals and finding out about any issues what will help by providing the support they need. guiding them to prioritise workloads, extra rest breaks. Individuals can also be signposted towards other people or organizations who may be able to give them support. With other people in the work or learning environment who know about the individual mental ill health, this is worrying for them, which case they should be supported.

Long-term support:

With long term Mental Health declines there is a serious Mental Health issue which individuals may need time off from work or learning. Which maybe they're not well enough to do the work they need to, or the medication there taking may cause drowsiness etc. Which they cannot carry out the

The Mind Matters ii:

work.

It's important to keep contact with the individual during their time off work or learning environment. They shouldn't be pressured to return. the contact should be positive and supporting, and not from a person who makes the individual feel part of the cause of anxiety or stress. Sending a get-well card just as they would with physical illness which also can be part of the contact. Occupational health specialists can assess the individual and suggest adjustments that may help the individual when they return to work.

Recovery:

Supporting individuals with Mental Ill Health, it's important to support recovery. recovery in Mental Health regards not as an absence of symptoms- everyone is on Mental health Continuum; symptoms may come and go- but development of resilience to cope with strains and stresses of everyday life.

From recovering in Mental Ill health is about individuals achieving personal goals and developing relationships and skills that support a positive approach to life, however or not they have ongoing mental health issues. Organizations can support recovery by encouraging and supporting strong relationships within the occupation, giving the individuals aspirations, goals that meet their hopes for the future.

Return to work:

An individual is returning to work following an absence due to mental ill health, they should feel supported.
A manager from the workplace should meet them before their return to discuss its organization's expectations and concerns they may have.

It should be decided from the individuals' preferences what colleagues will be told about their return and absence. Individuals could feel anxious and conscious about the return, with little things like meeting in the reception and arranging for them to have lunch with friendly colleague which can help them,

Their mental health should be kept monitored

Define the term person-centred.

A person-centred approach means that support and care is focused on the need of the individual rather

The Mind Matters ii:

that the organised around the support that the services can offer

Describe the importance of a person-centred approach for mental health.

1) It helps the individual to develop knowledge, skills- and confidence to make decisions about and to manage on their own support

2) Guidance and legislation require- person-centred approach and the personalisation of care services

3) Mental health professions have a responsibility to approach- care and support in person centred way

Now to look at the importance of recognising own responsibilities and limitations in relation to supporting the mental health of others.

Your responsibilities in the relation of supporting Mental Health will depend on your role in your organisation. If you're a tutor, manager or mentor for example, you may be trained to see the signs of mental ill health.
It's important to recognise your responsibility and

The Mind Matters ii:

limitations in the relation of supporting mental health of others so that you do not do anything that my cause harm to the individual or the organisation.
If you do not follow the adjustments that your organisation has put in place for an individual, you may risk the health of the individual and your own job role is best to always give a good reflection of the organisation rather than exposing the organisation to the risk of discrimination claim.

Each and everyone have a responsibility to treat people with respect in the workplace and to support colleagues

Let's Identify when it may be necessary to refer to others when supporting individuals with mental ill health.

Its best case is when the individual agrees to seek for help.
In this case you can refer them to an appropriate person or service. This individual cannot be persuaded to seek help for themselves. You might have to refer them if you think they may be at risk or possibly put others at risk, because of the wok they're doing.

*Refer individuals if!

The Mind Matters ii:

*If you think the individual is likely to harm themselves or is suicidal

*That you see signs of serious mental ill health such as psychosis but refuse to seek help for themselves.

*The individual could be doing something that could put other people at risk in becoming aggressive or violent towards others

You can call for help services NHS 111 OR 999   Individuals GP   Or qualified Mental Health First Aider if one is available in the organisation.

Explaining the role of the qualified mental health first aider.

They provide support for individuals who may be experiencing Mental Health issue or emotional distress,
Point of contact for any employee whose experiencing Mental Health issues including stress.
Which they are not trained Therapists but can recognise the signs of Mental Ill Health they listen and provide guidance.
Encouraging the individual to seek help, which

The Mind Matters ii:

may be from internal counselling services or external medical or counselling support, contacting emergency services if appropriate, maintaining appropriate levels of Confidentiality!

To Explain the importance of seeking support for own mental health.

Whilst supporting individuals with Mental ill health or who are distressed or going through stress at work, can also be stressful for the person supporting hem, if you're the one supporting the individual with Mental Health issues, then make sure you take care of yourself.

To Outline stigma and stereotypes relating to mental health illness.

The Stigma and Stereotypes can usually mean that individuals are labelled differently and in a negative way, this stigma arises from the misconceptions that people may have about Mental Health Illness. These Misconceptions come from the lack of knowledge that they have about Mental Health among the general public.

Describing how attitudes and perceptions can influence an individual with mental ill health.

The public attitudes and perceptions can lead to stereotyping of individuals with Mental Health conditions as dangerous an unpredictable, which can lead them to be socially excluded and also become isolated from the community, which can turn its cause into a further deterioration within their Mental Health. The **Prejudice** is where people hold opinions about those with Mental Health conditions, which can affect the way that individuals are treated.
The discrimination is where individuals are treated differently due to their Mental Health condition. Maybe they're not offered a job because of it or are excluded from activities. Sometimes it's easily excused how somebody can treat another in the terms of bullying

Summarise Outline stigma and stereotypes relating to mental health:

The Stigma and Stereotypes can usually mean that individuals are labelled differently and in a negative way, this stigma arises from the misconceptions that people may have about Menta Health Illness. These Misconceptions come from the lack of knowledge that they have about Mental Health among the public. You have to remember people

The Mind Matters ii:

who haven't suffered from Mental Health trauma will not acknowledge those who suffer a distraction from what they may deem as normality, other Mental Health suffering can still excel in many different hobbies or interests, Such as athleticism, keyboard, pianoist, guitarist

but disclose their Mental Health Illness. What defines how bad someone's Mental Health Illness is defined to what the Health Professional diagnosis of what antagonizing their symptoms from, their daily living life, so it's very rude of other individuals to manipulate their quality and make them a victim of bullying.

Describing how attitudes and perceptions can influence an individual with mental ill health.

The public attitudes and perceptions can lead to stereotyping of individuals with Mental Health conditions as dangerous an unpredictable, which can lead them to be socially excluded and also become isolated from the community, which can turn its cause into a further deterioration within their Mental Health. The **Prejudice** is where people hold opinions about those with Mental Health conditions, which can affect the way that individuals are treated.
The discrimination is where individuals are treated differently due to their Mental Health condition.

The Mind Matters ii:

Maybe they're not offered a job because of it or are excluded from activities

Let's Summarise the impact media can have on an individual's mental health and well-being.

It's past stigma with people with Mental Health illnesses it was commonly portrayed within the media as dangerous and violent, with a disturbed thoughtful process and unpredictable behaviour. The media has played a role in its spreading of these myth's about Mental Illness, (Such as horror movies about the 'psycho' killers) escaping from 'The Metropolitan Lunatic Asylum'.

Today modern media embraces the importance of equality and diversity, which has helped to minimize prejudice and fear amongst its wider populace, this give a prodigious impact on Mental Ill Health.

The Media has a huge impact on a lot of people's feelings-thoughts and self-image, These negative images of mental ill health can have an impact, which leaving some individuals feeling shamed and distressed about their condition.
Glam, models and celebrities, can leave individuals feeling inadequate and distressed.
Most of these Stars like to conform to ideals of

The Mind Matters ii:

what society expects to look like this, but truth is majority of people don't look like this.

Explaining how mental ill health can impact;

Which Can lead to individuals feeling inferior and having a negative self-image, intense feelings of self-hate, anger or disgust and uselessness. Physical health can also be affected by high blood pressure, lack of sleep and unhealthy eating as the individual fails to take care of themselves.

Family, friends, and colleagues:

Ill Mental Health can affect even basic interactions with family, friends and colleagues, some individuals experiencing mental health problems find it difficult to nurture relationships and have problems with commitment or intimacy, or frequent encounter sexual health problems.

Learning/education:

The importance of understanding egalitarian as everyone deserves equal rights and opportunities, it's important to offer people who suffer from mental

ill health or mental health, some support, guidance so they don't feel or become isolated.
The individuals who live with mental ill health may socially isolate themselves and develop anxiety and concentration problems, which can affect their access to educational opportunities and their inclusion to success in educational learning.

Work/employment:

Mental health conditions may make it more difficult for individuals to engage with the workplace activities and colleagues, meet and manage deadlines, also manage their own roles at work.

Day to day living

Preparing meals, getting dressed, personal hygiene, cleaning of the house, looking after children and working schedule can be more difficult for those with Mental Ill Health., This may be a time when finances are reduced due to absence from employment and can leap into financial difficulty.

Identify relevant legislation and guidance in relation to mental health provision.

The Mind Matters ii:

Mental Health Legislation is an area of Law that applies to the people who received a diagnosis or potential diagnosis of Mental illness.

There is two specific pieces of legislation that apply to whom have Mental Health problems. Which are:

;Mental Health act 1983-2007   : Mental Capacity act 2005

The key bits of legislation will impact on individual experiencing Mental Illness are Health and Social Care Act 2008 and the Care Act 2014. Which they provide framework for the provision of care of all individuals who require it.

Health and Social Care Act 2008 set up the regulation of Adult Health and Social Care Services to ensure that service users receive safe care!

The care Act 2014 works on the improvement of independence and well-being for individuals through to provision of joined up person-centred. Health and Care Services.

Identifying drivers in relation to mental health provision.

The National Health Services (NHS)

The Mind Matters ii:

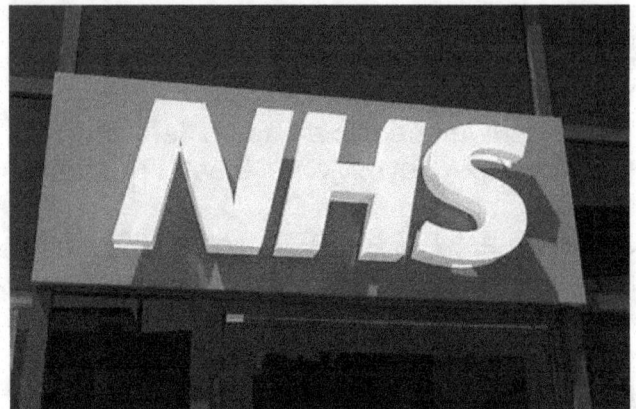

Major provider of healthcare including Mental Health through GP's. Hospital Specialists Mental Health Services, Providing Services the NHS collects Data on the numbers of Mental Health Patients seen.

Joseph Rowntree Foundation;
An independent social change organisation, are primarily concerned with addressing poverty. Also concerning about Mental Health because Mental Ill Health can arise from the cause of poverty, which they provide reports on issues related to poverty.

Describing how policy can support the mental health of individuals.

Mental Health Policies support Mental Health by setting up benchmarks and co-ordinating the

The Mind Matters ii:

Government objectives for Mental Health, Policy, supported by legislation of which sets up the framework then by which the provisions are delivered, and individuals should benefit from co-ordinated of quality supports for Mental Health.

Describe strategies to promote well-being.

Giving individuals greater control- over learning their work or learning

Involving individual- in decision making

training line managers- or tutors to ensure the can support the delegation of control and decision making

Promote good leadership and good -m Relationships between leaders in the organisation

Reducing stress and early intervention for Mental Health is - An important factor in improving well-being.

Outline sources of information, resources and support for mentally healthy environments;

The Mind Matters ii:

Internal sources:

Mental Health first aiders appointed in the work/learning environment.

Mental Health Champions

Internal counsellors

Trade Union and staff Association support

External sources:

The World Health Organization.
The Health and Safety executive
Charitable organisation such as mind and the Mental health Foundation.
Government organisations, The office for Mental Health improvement and disparities

Identify strategies to reduce barriers to accessing mental health support.

The stigma of Mental Ill Health- concerns about confidentiality and trust.
Concerns about being seen as

The Mind Matters ii:

weak or incapable- dislike, talking about Mental Health problems believing the problem is not serious enough to ask for help- Not having easy access to Health Professionals who can help. being able to take time away from work for an appointment-Concerns about the treatments that may be offered and their impact.

Concerned about what others will think- fears about the outcome of seeking help- language barriers where individuals don't speak English as a first language and may not be able to express themselves.

Talking about Mental Health to address the misconceptions developing a knowledge and awareness of Mental Health issues.

Encouraging individuals to seek early help in the knowledge that this could prevent more serious Mental Ill Health- making it clear individuals can access help in the organisation.

Emphasising that no problem is two significant to talk about individuals to identify the early signs of stress and Mental ill Health.
Ensuring confidentiality around Mental Ill Health matter to build trust- creating safe environments where individuals do not fear the consequences of admitting to Mental Health issues.

Making environments and information accessible to speakers of other languages by using

The Mind Matters ii:

translators and printed leaflets in other languages-understanding and working to challenge different cultural perceptions of Mental ill Health.

Looking into the importance of promoting mentally healthy environments in the workplace.

It's important because mental ill health in the UK accounts for some 70 million lost working days each year mentally healthy environments reduce absenteeism but also productivity and performance in the workplace, a happier workplace is also more able to cope with change or difficult situations. The reputation of the organisation is improved as well as the physical Health of employees then the organisation will meet their legal responsibilities

Defining what is meant by a wellness action plan.

A wellness action plan is a confidential document that is agreed between the employer or manager within the organisation and employee to identify what will protect the employee's Mental Health and well-being at work. Every employee should have a wellness action plan whether they have an existing Health problem or not,

The Mind Matters ii:

The importance of a wellness action plan for self and others.

-It starts the conversation about Mental Health and sets out the expectations of employees and employers. It's a proactive approach to managing mental health at work rather than a reactive approach, so it anticipates what could go wrong and puts safeguarding in place to prevent or reduce the risk rather than dealing with the impact of mental health issues once it arises..

A wellness action plan is a confidential doc that is agreed between employer or manager within the organisation and employee to identify what will protect the employee's Mental health and well-being at work. Every employee should have a wellness action plan weather they have an existing health problem or not.

Identify key components of a wellness action plan.

Giving examples that an individual can use to support their Mental well-being. Contains examples of signs or symptoms or stress or mental ill health that can then alert the employer, any triggers in the workplace are identified.
highlights any potential impacts of stress or mental ill health on the individual performance

The Mind Matters ii:

Let's preform an wellness action plan for individuals that may help support a better Mental health at work or in a relationship, with the benefit of ideas; Understanding our individual want or need at work weather that be cutting down the working hours, working solely in a segregated room away from others or guidance from another individual that relates to your health and wellbeing, performing work perhaps with headphones on can sometimes boost your morale. Building a relationship with friends that can adjust to your wants and needs, someone who can listen, who understands your frustration, you may find counselling works well for you, or you may find them more daunting to have the discussion of how they can support you further, but usually they can have access for different ideas and institutions that may better your wellbeing to become accepted as an individual that suffers from Mental Health or Mental Ill health, a neurologist and phycologist can preform a variety of tasks that you can either adjust with a variety of cognitive skills tests which you can work well with or struggle with, such as number puzzle, remember shapes and sentences this can give a focus on your skill sets. Many modern Mobile Phone devices have app stores which you can download app to better your memory and task the skills you want to benefit from, crosswords, sudoku and many, many more.

The Mind Matters ii:

Tips for Health and Nutrition Based on Evidence

Limit sugary beverages.

The main source of added sugar in the American diet is sweetened beverages including soda, fruit juices, and tea.

Unfortunately, research indicates that even in those who do not have excess body fat, drinking sugar-sweetened beverages increases the risk of type 2 diabetes and heart disease. Sugar-sweetened beverages are particularly detrimental for kids since they can cause illnesses including type 2 diabetes, high blood pressure, and non-alcoholic fatty liver disease, which typically do not manifest in children until maturity.

The high fat content of nuts causes some people to shun them. But seeds and nuts are highly nourishing. They include a tonne of protein, fibre, and other vitamins and minerals. Nuts may aid with weight loss and lower your risk of heart disease and type 2 diabetes. One significant observational study also found that a low diet of nuts and seeds may be associated with an increased risk of death from heart disease, stroke, or type 2 diabetes.

The Mind Matters ii:

Skip the highly processed meals.

Foods with ingredients that have undergone extensive modification from their original state are considered ultra-processed. Added sugar, highly refined oil, salt, preservatives, artificial sweeteners, colours, and flavours are among the additives that are frequently included in them.

Examples comprise:

cake snacks

swift food

frozen food

meals in cans chips

Ultra-processed foods are highly delicious, which makes them easy to overeat, and they activate reward-related brain regions, which might result in an excessive intake of calories and weight gain. According to studies, eating a lot of ultra-processed food can increase your risk of developing chronic diseases like type 2 diabetes, heart disease, and obesity.

They typically contain low-quality components including processed carbohydrates, inflammatory fats, and added sugar in addition to being deficient in fibre, protein, and minerals. They primarily offer empty calories as a result.

The Mind Matters ii:

Have no fear of coffee

Despite some disagreement, coffee has a tonne of health advantages.

Because of its high antioxidant content, coffee consumption has been associated in some studies to longer life expectancy, a lower risk of type 2 diabetes, Parkinson's and Alzheimer's diseases, as well as a host of other disorders.

The recommended daily intake seems to be between three and four cups, however pregnant women should limit or avoid it entirely because it has been associated to low birth weight.

Coffee and other products with caffeine should be consumed in moderation, though. Consuming too much caffeine can cause heart palpitations and insomnia, among other health problems. Limit your daily consumption of coffee to no more than four cups, and stay away from high-calorie, high-sugar additives like sweetened creamer.

ingest oily fish

A fantastic source of high-quality protein and good fat is fish. This is especially true of fatty fish like salmon, which are rich in anti-inflammatory omega-3 fatty acids and other minerals.

The Mind Matters ii:

According to studies, those who frequently consume fish had a lower risk of developing a number of diseases, such as heart disease, dementia, and inflammatory bowel disease.

Obtain enough rest.

It is impossible to stress the significance of obtaining adequate good sleep.

Insufficient sleep can worsen insulin resistance, mess with your hormones that control appetite, and lower both your physical and mental function.

Additionally, a weak individual risk factor for weight growth and obesity is getting too little sleep. Lack of sleep influences a person's tendency to choose foods richer in fat, sugar, and calories, which may result in unintended weight gain.

aliment your gut flora

The gut microbiota, a term that refers to all of the microorganisms in your gut, is crucial for overall health. Obesity and a variety of digestive issues are among the chronic diseases that have been related to a change in gut flora. Consuming probiotic foods like yoghurt and sauerkraut, supplementing with probiotics when necessary, and eating a lot of fibre are all effective

The Mind Matters ii:

approaches to enhance gut health. Notably, fibre provides your gut flora with a prebiotic, or food supply.

Keep hydrated.

Hydration is a crucial yet frequently disregarded indicator of health. Staying hydrated ensures that your body is operating at its peak efficiency and that your blood volume is enough.

The best approach to stay hydrated is to drink water, which has no calories, sugar, or chemicals. Although there isn't a specific quantity that everyone requires each day, try to drink enough to sufficiently quench your thirst.

Eat only lightly browned meats.

Meat can be a wholesome and nutritious component of your diet. It is a great source of nutrients and is highly high in protein.

But when meat is burned or charred, issues arise. The development of hazardous substances as a result of this charring may raise your chance of developing certain malignancies.

Avoid burning or charring the meat when cooking it. Limit your diet of red and processed meats as well, such as bacon and lunch meat, because they raise your risk of colon cancer and general cancer.

The Mind Matters ii:

Before going to bed, avoid bright lighting.

In the evening, exposure to strong lights that emit blue light wavelengths may interfere with your body's ability to produce the hormone melatonin, which promotes sleep.

Wearing blue light-blocking eyewear can help you decrease your exposure to blue light, especially if you spend a lot of time in front of a computer or other digital screen. You should also avoid using digital devices for 30 to 60 minutes before bed.

As night-time draws in, this may improve your body's natural melatonin production, promoting sounder sleep.

If you're lacking, take vitamin D.

Vitamin D intake is typically inadequate. Although this widespread vitamin D deficiency are not immediately hazardous, maintaining appropriate vitamin D levels can assist to improve bone density, lessen depressive symptoms, boost immune function, and reduce cancer risk.

Your vitamin D levels may be low if you do not spend a lot of time outdoors.

It's a good idea to get your levels checked if you can, so you can adjust them if necessary, by taking vitamin D supplements.

The Mind Matters ii:

Consume a lot of fruit and veggies.

Prebiotic fibre, vitamins, minerals, and antioxidants, many of which have powerful health benefits, are abundant in fruits and vegetables.

According to studies, people who consume more fruits and vegetables live longer and are at a decreased risk of developing heart disease, obesity, and other diseases.

Consume enough protein.

Consuming adequate protein will help you stay healthy since it gives your body the building blocks it needs to make new cells and tissues.

Additionally, this substance is crucial for maintaining a healthy body weight.

While making you feel full, a high protein diet may increase your metabolic rate, or rate at which calories are burned. Additionally, it might make you feel less compelled to eat late-night snacks.

Make a move

One of the best things you can do for your mental and physical health is to engage in aerobic exercise, or cardio.

The Mind Matters ii:

It works especially well at shedding belly fat, the unhealthy kind of fat that collects around your organs. Your metabolic health may significantly improve as a result of less abdominal fat.

The Physical Activity Guidelines for Citizens recommend that we aim for at least 150 minutes a week of low intensity exercise.

Don't use drugs or smoke, and only consume alcohol in moderation.

Abuse of alcohol, illegal drug usage, and smoking can all have detrimental effects on your health.

If you engage in any of these behaviours, you might want to scale back or stop to lower your chance of developing chronic illnesses.

To assist with this, there are services online and perhaps in your neighbourhood as well. To find out more about obtaining resources, speak with your doctor.

Make use of extra virgin olive oil.

One of the healthiest vegetable oils you may use is extra virgin olive oil. Heart-healthy

The Mind Matters ii:

monounsaturated fats and potent antioxidants with anti-inflammatory qualities are abundant in it.

According to some data, extra virgin olive oil may be good for the heart because those who eat it have a lower risk of dying from heart attacks and strokes.

Reduce your sugar consumption.

Modern foods and beverages frequently contain added sugar. High consumption is associated with type 2 diabetes, heart disease, and obesity.

The World Health Organization advises reducing added sugars to 5% or fewer of your daily calories for optimal health, whereas the Dietary Guidelines for Americans advise keeping added sugar intake below 10% of your daily calorie intake.

Limit your intake of processed carbohydrates.

Carbs are not all made equal.

Refined carbohydrates lack fibre because of their intensive processing. They contain relatively few nutrients and, when consumed in excess, may be harmful to your health. The majority of ultra-processed foods are created with refined carbohydrates such white flour, processed corn, and added sugars.

According to studies, consuming a lot of refined carbohydrates may lead to overeating, weight gain, and chronic conditions like type 2 diabetes and heart disease.

Lift hefty objects

One of the best types of exercise to build your muscles and enhance your body composition is strength and resistance training.

It may also result in significant benefits in metabolic health, such as better insulin sensitivity, which makes it simpler to control blood sugar levels, and increases in metabolic rate, which refers to how many calories you burn while at rest.

If you don't have weights, you can produce resistance with your own bodyweight or with the use of resistance bands to obtain a similar workout with many of the same advantages.

The Physical Avoid synthetic trans fats.

Artificial trans fats are unhealthy man-made fats that have a strong association with heart disease and inflammation.

The Mind Matters ii:

Since they are now totally prohibited in the US and many other nations, avoiding them should be considerably simpler. Keep in mind that some foods may still contain trace levels of naturally occurring trans fats, but these are not as harmful as trans fats produced artificially. American Activity Guidelines advises

Utilize several herbs and spices

Today, more than ever, we have access to a wide selection of herbs and spices. In addition to flavour, they might also provide a number of health advantages.

As an illustration, the powerful anti-inflammatory and antioxidant properties of ginger and turmeric may aid to improve your general health.

You should strive to include a wide variety of herbs and spices in your diet due to their significant potential health advantages.

Maintain your interpersonal connections.

Social connections with close friends, relatives, and other people you care about are crucial for both your emotional and physical health.

The Mind Matters ii:

According to studies, persons who have close friends and family tend to live longer and in better health.

periodically keeping a food journal

Since calculating your portion sizes and calorie intake is not inaccurate, the only way to know exactly how many calories you consume is to measure your food and use a nutrition tracker.

Your consumption of protein, fibre, and micronutrients can be better understood with the help of tracking.

There is some data that suggests those who track their food intake are more successful at losing weight and keeping it off, despite several research linking tracking calories and disordered eating behaviours.

Remove more belly fat

An increased risk of cardiometabolic disorders including type 2 diabetes and heart disease is associated with excessive abdominal fat, also known as visceral fat.

The Mind Matters ii:

Because of this, your waist size and waist-to-hip ratio may be significantly more accurate indicators of your health than your weight.

Cutting back on refined carbohydrates, increasing your intake of protein and fibre, and lowering your stress levels (which can lower cortisol, a stress hormone that promotes the build-up of abdominal fat) are all methods that may help you lose belly fat.

Remove more belly fat

Avoid following strict diets

Diets rarely produce long-lasting results and are typically ineffectual. Dieting in the past is among the best indicators of future weight gain.

This is since excessively restricted diets decrease your metabolic rate, or the number of calories you burn each day, which makes it more challenging to lose weight. Additionally, they change your satiety and hunger hormones, making you feel hungrier and possibly inducing intense food cravings for meals heavy in fat, calories, and sugar.

All of this might lead to "yo-yo" dieting or rebound weight gain. Remove more belly fat

The Mind Matters ii:

Avoid following strict diets

Diets rarely produce long-lasting results and are typically ineffectual. Dieting in the past is among the best indicators of future weight gain.

This is because excessively restricted diets decrease your metabolic rate, or the number of calories you burn each day, which makes it more challenging to lose weight. Additionally, they change your satiety and hunger hormones, making you feel hungrier and possibly inducing intense food cravings for meals heavy in fat, calories, and sugar.

This is all a recipe for whole eggs.

Although the topic of eggs and health is frequently debated, it is a fallacy that eggs are unhealthy due of their high cholesterol level. Studies reveal that they are a fantastic source of protein and nutrients and have little to no impact on blood cholesterol in the majority of people.

In addition, an analysis comprising 263,938 individuals discovered no correlation between egg consumption and the risk of heart disease or for "yoyo" dieting, or the tendency to regain lost weight.

The Mind Matters ii:

Meditate

Your health is negatively impacted by stress. Blood sugar levels, eating preferences, disease propensity, weight, fat distribution, and other factors can all be impacted. Therefore, it's crucial to learn effective stress management techniques.

One such method is meditation, which has some scientific backing for its utility in reducing stress and enhancing health.

Researchers showed that meditation reduced LDL (bad) cholesterol and inflammation in one trial of 48 individuals with high blood pressure, type 2 diabetes, or both when compared to the control group. The participants in the meditation group also reported greater bodily and emotional wellness.

The conclusion

You're eating habits and wellness can be greatly enhanced by taking a few easy measures. However, if you want to live a better life, don't just concentrate on your diet. Additionally crucial are social interactions, sleep, and exercise. With the following evidence-based advice, it's simple to make minor adjustments that can have a significant effect on your general health.

Let's focus on some simple ideas of home exercises;

1. Bear Crawl

Sets: 4 | Reps: 5 – 10 (4 steps forward and back equates to 1 rep)

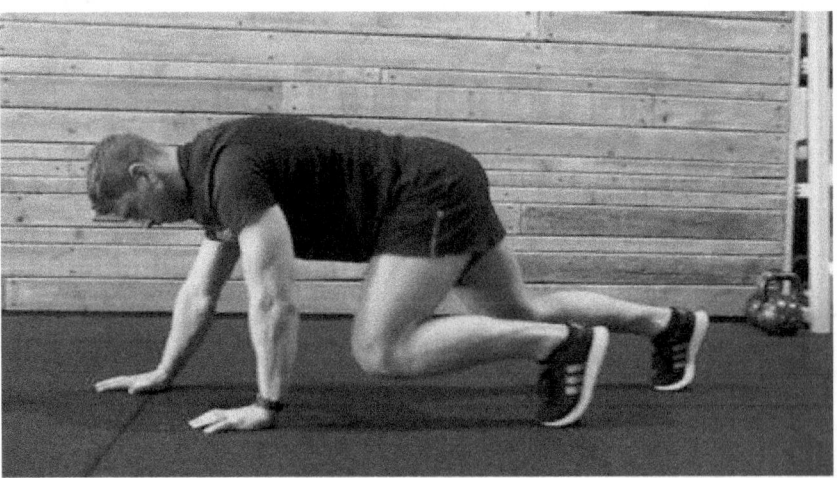

One of my all-time favourite exercises using only body weight is this. There will be specific attention paid to your shoulders and abs, but no muscle will go unused.

Start with your knees about three inches off the ground and your hands beneath your shoulders.

Simply advance your left hand and right foot together for a short distance before repeating on the other side.

You should concentrate on fully contracting your abs with each forward or backward step to keep your hips from rotating.

Keep your breath steady throughout this action.

2. Squat Jump

Sets: 4 | Reps: 15 – 20

An old favourite to condition those legs and elevate your heart rate. You'll hit your quads and glutes with this but be sure to keep your heels down when you squat to stop your calves having all the fun.

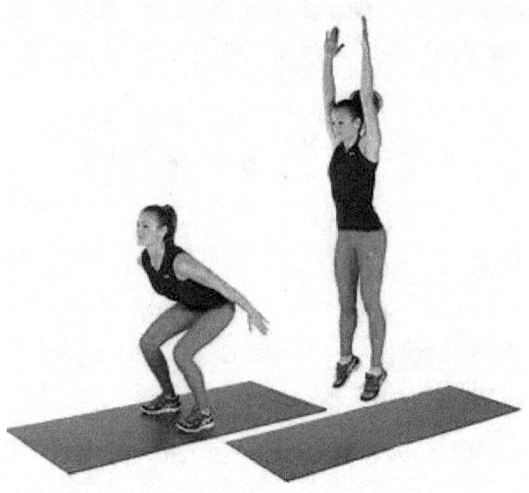

Start with your feet somewhat wider than hip-width apart (whichever feels more comfortable)

If you can't squat much lower without bending at the lower back, squat till your thighs are parallel to the ground.

Standing up from the bottom of the squat, push your feet off the ground with as much force as you can

Keep your eyes forward while raising your chest.

When you land, flex your knees to lessen the impact, then immediately start the next rep.

Regression: Just do a bodyweight squat without the jump.

The Mind Matters ii:

3. Maximum of 4 Press Up Sets and Reps (with good technique)

Sometimes there is simply no need to create something entirely new. This is a fundamental exercise for both novice and expert home exercises. Working mostly the chest and triceps, with a little bit of bite developing in the shoulders as you complete more reps.

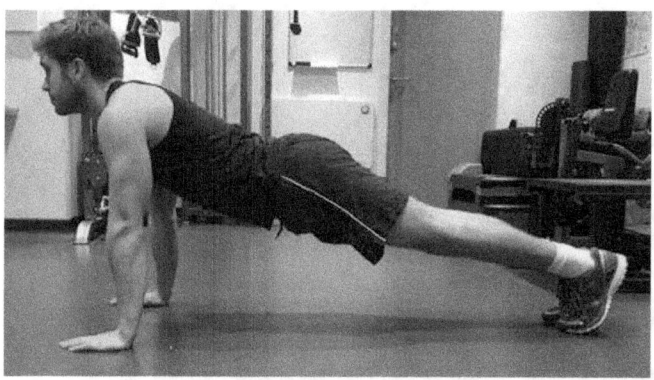

With your abs contracted and your hands right outside your shoulders (make sure you are not arching your lower back and dropping your hips)

The Mind Matters ii:

Remember that it's how low your chest goes, not how high your nose, so that your shoulders are parallel to your elbows or just a little lower.

By pushing through the heel of your hand and consciously contracting your chest, you can get back to the starting posture.

Regression: To make this easier, get on your knees and constrict your range of motion to match your strength.

4. Jump Lunges: 4 Sets | 10–20 Reps

Bring it with you on this one. It can cause you to collapse at the hips and bounce your chest off your thigh. When done properly, you'll increase your heart rate and effectively work your glutes.

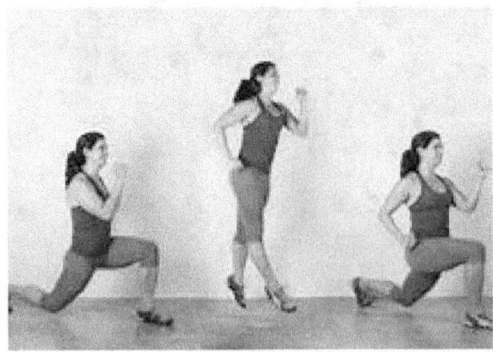

The Mind Matters ii:

Step back with your back leg bent until your front thigh is parallel to the ground.

Drive your feet off the ground and forcefully drive them into the floor.

Keep your gaze forward and your chest raised.

Quickly and precisely change your stance in the air, then kneel upon landing.

Stop letting your chest drop toward your thigh by engaging your abs.

Continue with steps 2 through 5 for each leg until you have finished all of your reps.

Regression: Substitute a forward- or backward-stepping lunge for the jump (see the dumbbell version of this in the Home Dumbbell exercises section below)

5. 4 sets; 5–10 repetitions.

I hear you asking, "How can I possible include this exercise in a beginner's routine." Simply told, it's one of the most efficient, calorie-dense, and adaptable exercises you can perform at home. from your back knee to your front thigh.

The Mind Matters ii:

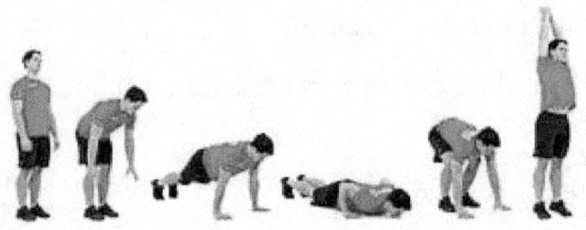

Put your hands on the ground and bend only your knees, not your back.

Return your feet to a complete plank position by jumping or walking.

Lay your chest on the ground.

Jump your feet inwards and return to a complete plank.

Drive hard into the ground, then leap as high as you can.

When you land, bend your knees, and start the following rep right away.

Regression: During the press, maintain your knees lowered and step your feet out and in. Simply omit tip number 5 and push yourself to your personal boundaries if the jumps leave you reaching for the sick pail.

The Mind Matters ii:

6. 3 sets per leg. 10 to 15 times per leg.

When you start filling up your swimsuit with well-defined curves in the summer, you'll be happy you started this training regimen. With some assistance from your quads, your glutes will be where you feel this the most. Important: Avoid over-bouncing off your back foot to prevent your calves from taking over.

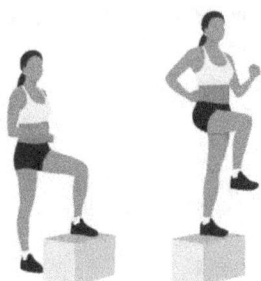

Step one flat foot onto your bench or chair.

The Mind Matters ii:

To avoid flailing your arms and building momentum, keep your hands in front at chest level.

Standing tall, elevating your chest, and keeping your eyes forward, shift your weight to your front leg.

Back off and keep your foot firmly planted on the chair.

To avoid bouncing on your rear foot when doing the next rep, pause for a little moment before doing so.

Perform complete repetitions on one leg before switching.

Progress - By using the first or second step of your staircase or your sofa, you can reduce the height of your step-up. To further lower the height, take out the sofa cushions.

7. Bench Dips, 4 sets, 10 to 15 repetitions

Most people won't end up looking like those athletes who can hover in between reps while clapping their hands behind their back when they

The Mind Matters ii:

properly perform press-ups; instead, they may end up face planting on the carpet. To begin developing strength in your triceps, chest, and shoulders, try the bench dip.

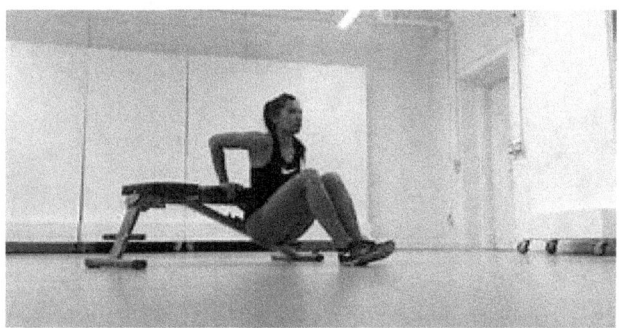

Put your hands on the bench or chair slightly outside your hips.

bent knees with your feet forward (the greater the bend the easier it will be)

until your upper arm is parallel to the floor, bring your hips down (or as far as you can comfortably go)

Your hips should remain close to the bench.

Activate your hand's heel and raise your arms.

Consider holding for a split second at the peak while tightening your triceps.

The Mind Matters ii:

Regression: You can make this exercise easier to complete by limiting your range of motion and bending your knees more.

8. Toe taps: 4 sets of 20–30 repetitions.

How can you make running on the spot more precise and poised? Give me your toes, please. This will undoubtedly increase your heart rate because it makes you elevate your foot higher than if you were just running on the spot. This is a fantastic addition to any at-home workout because it engages your abs slightly while working almost all of the muscles in your lower body.

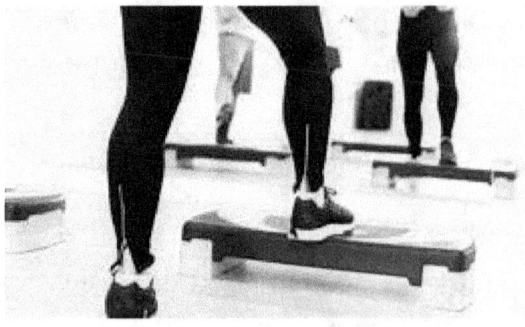

Place one foot's toes on the bench and maintain your whole weight on the leg that is on the ground.

The Mind Matters ii:

Just enough of a bounce off the rear foot to lift off the ground

Quickly and precisely change your feet.

As you would if you were sprinting on the spot, your goal is to complete each rep with no breaks.

Maintain an elevated chest and continue to breathe.

Regression: If you're just starting off, you might need to slow down a little bit while trying to move your feet quickly and simultaneously.

9. Split Squat with Back Leg Raised (112 Reps)

3 sets per leg. 8 to 12 times on each leg.

There is absolutely no way to cheat, thus I have no doubt that this will test your leg strength. It depends greatly on your posture and body position where you feel the exercise working your glutes, hamstrings, and quadriceps the most.

The Mind Matters ii:

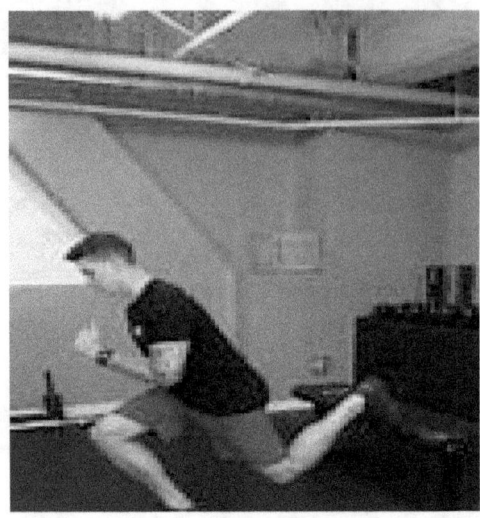

Take a medium step forward with your back to the bench, raising your back foot onto the seat.

You can stand up straight without your lower back arching excessively. Straighten your back and slightly lean forward if you detect this.

Lower your rear knee while bending your front leg. When pressing upward, pay attention to pushing against the front foot's heel.

Every full rep should be followed by a half rep, making a complete rep out of 1 full and 1 half rep.

The Mind Matters ii:

Perform complete repetitions on one leg before switching.

Regression: Try this initially with both feet on the ground if it feels awkward or too difficult.

10. Shoulder Press: 4 Sets, 8–12 Reps.

This crucial exercise, which may be done standing or seated, is necessary to increase shoulder strength. Your triceps will hold your shoulders as you reach the top of the push, working primarily the middle and fronts of your shoulders.

The Mind Matters ii:

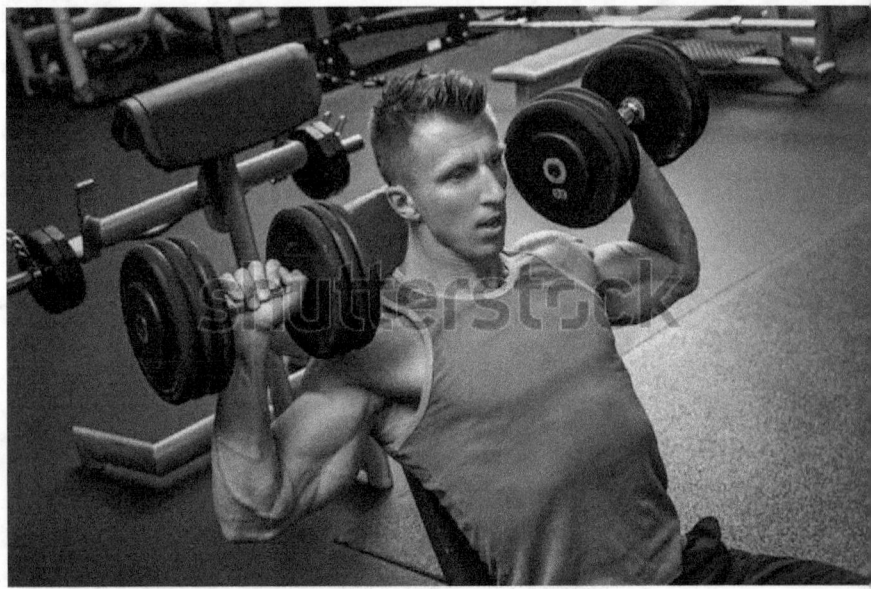

Whether you're standing or sitting, begin with the dumbbells under your shoulders.

As your flexibility permits, raise the dumbbells overhead until your arms are fully extended.

Control-fully and without letting them rest on your shoulders, return the dumbbells.

Allow yourself to maintain a straight back and resist the urge to do so.

Regression: Try to go with a lighter weight. Focus on bent-over rows and press-ups to develop a stronger foundation if your weight options are limited and this isn't a possibility.

The Mind Matters ii:

The Mind Matters ii: